THE CARE BOOK

A planning & resource guide to support your journey
from accidental to intentional caregiving

DR. KIMBERLY FRASER RN, PHD

SUTHERLAND
HOUSE

TORONTO, 2023

Sutherland House
416 Moore Ave., Suite 205
Toronto, ON M4G 1C9

First edition, October 2023

If you are interested in inviting one of our authors to a live event or
media appearance, please contact sranasinghe@sutherlandhousebooks.com
and visit our website at sutherlandhousebooks.com for more
information about our authors and their schedules.

We acknowledge the support of the Government of Canada.

Manufactured in Canada
Cover designed by Jordan Lunn
Book composed by Karl Hunt

Library and Archives Canada Cataloguing in Publication
Title: The care book : a planning and resource guide to support your journey
from accidental to intentional caregiving / Kimberly Fraser.
Names: Fraser, Kimberly, author.
Identifiers: Canadiana 20230538223 | ISBN 9781990823756 (softcover)
Subjects: LCSH: Caregivers—Handbooks, manuals, etc. | LCGFT: Handbooks and manuals.
Classification: LCC RA645.3 .F735 2023 | DDC 362.14—dc23

ISBN 978-1-990823-75-6

The Care Book

A planning and resource to support your journey
from accidental to intentional caregiving

This resource guide will be with the care recipient when you can't be. It provides useful and important information to others who may be involved with the care of your family member or friend. It will assist others to provide care, meet personal needs, and solve problems so that those helping with care, or covering for you, can provide compassionate and informed care like you do.

THIS CARE BOOK IS ABOUT _____.

You may choose to attach
a photo of the care
recipient here

Dedicated to all past, present, and future caregivers.

*May you always have the necessary tools and information
to support you in any caregiving role.*

CONTENTS

CONTENTS

INTRODUCTION

You may have read my book *The Accidental Caregiver: Wisdom and guidance for the unexpected challenges of family caregiving,* or perhaps not. Regardless, this guidebook, also known as the Care Book, was a natural extension of The Accidental Caregiver. Information sourcing, tracking and organizing is a daunting chore for many family caregivers. They consistently told me that in my research studies, when I engaged with them as a director of a large home care organization, and frankly, nearly every time I talked to someone who was providing care to a friend or loved one.

Whereas *The Accidental Caregiver*, a narrative of the challenges and triumphs experienced by the people whose stories I share in the book, and contains many ideas, tips, and guidelines , the Care Book you are holding is specific to the loved one YOU are caring for. Not only are there ideas and suggestions about the kind of information to gather, store, and use in the care, it organizes the information in a user friendly manner. It can be regularly updated. It can be shared with others who are involved with the care and support of your friend or loved one so you, the primary family caregiver, does not need to keep all that information in your head to share with one person at a time. You can give access to The Care Book to any one you feel needs the information.

Keeping information up to date and in one place supports continuity of care because anyone involved in the care and support can see what is being done, review instructions and guidelines, and document anything they have done. It is all in one place–in The Care Book.

What is the Care Book and why have a Care Book?

This guidebook is intended to support your information management and care planning as a family caregiver. Your role is instrumental to the health and well-being of the loved one or friend for whom you are caring. This is a convenient place to keep all of the pertinent information related to their health and social needs, important contacts and phone numbers, as well as daily and weekly care needs and instructions. It also has additional templates for you to copy for documenting care and activities.

How to use the Care Book?

I suggest you initially read through the Care Book to get a feel for the various sections and think about how you might use it. Some family caregivers write in the Care Book as is and share it openly with others coming into provide care–other family and friends, paid providers, and even bring it to facilities to share in the case of respite stays out of the home. Others copy the forms and templates they want to use and create a separate binder. They then share the binder with others, while keeping the original as a master copy in a private area of the home. It is entirely up to you to decide how you will use the various resources in this book.

You will note that some sections are helpful now, some may be helpful in the future, and some you may wish to modify to suit your particular situation.

The pages at the beginning of this book are forms for you to fill out–helpful information and contacts about the person you are caring for. You may wish to do this in pencil so you can update accordingly.

After the forms, there are sample pages so that those caring for your friend or loved one can document what they did that day, the medications and treatments given, and a place for them to write daily notes for you. These pages might be used for other family or unpaid caregivers who assist in the care from time to time or during periods of respite for you, or perhaps private care providers you hire and pay a fee to.

It is also helpful if you want any providers who come in from a local home care program to provide care to leave you notes of what they have done. Many home care programs or agencies may have their own notes that are left in the home and you can read those, but in cases where they do not leave documentation you have the right to request that they document their activities in your Care Book as well. Documentation supports open communication and consistent care for your loved one.

All of the forms and templates throughout the book are duplicated in the Forms and Templates section for you to copy as needed.

About

ABOUT _____ ALSO LIKES TO BE CALLED _____

Primary Family Caregiver Name: _____

Primary Caregiver Contact: _____

Special Dates and People: _____

_____

_____

Children/Grandchildren and special notes:_____

_____

Close friends/family and usual visitors:_____

_____

Hobbies and Interests: _____

Likes and Dislikes: _____

Proud Moments/Occupation/Jobs/Memberships/Places Lived: _____

_____

_____

_____

_____

Favorite topics of conversation: _____

_____

Food Preferences

BREAKFAST		
Usual		
Special Occasions/Treats		
LUNCH		
Usual		
Special Occasions/Treats		
SUPPER/DINNER		
Usual		
Special Occasions/Treats		
GENERAL	**FAVORITES**	**DISLIKES**
Vegetables		
Fruits		
Beverages		
Snacks/Treats		

Other notes: _____

_____

_____

_____

*This information was updated on_____.

4

About the Diagnoses or Conditions
(Strengths and Areas of Support)

Diagnosis/Conditions: _____

_____

_____

_____

_____

_____

_____

_____

_____

Areas of particular strengths: _____

_____

_____

Areas of specific supports:_____

_____

_____

_____

Allergies

ALLERGIC TO:	WHAT HAPPENS:	HOW TO TREAT:

What to do in case of emergency: _____

_____

_____

_____

_____

_____

_____

Other important things to know about: _____

_____

_____

_____

_____

_____

*This information was updated on_____.

Daily Schedule At-a-Glance

AM _____

_____

NOON _____

_____

PM _____

_____

EVENING _____

_____

Weekly Schedule At-a-Glance

TIME (AM/PM)	MON	TUES	WED	THURS	FRI	SAT	SUN

Notes: _____

_____

*This information was updated on_____.

Self-care Needs
(Abilities and Assistance required)

Activities of Daily Living

Date revised: _____

BATHING/SHOWERING	FEEDING
❑ Independent ❑ Partial Assistance ❑ Full Assistance Special Instructions:	❑ Independent ❑ Partial Assistance ❑ Full Assistance Special Instructions:
DRESSING GROOMING	TOILETING
❑ Independent ❑ Partial Assistance ❑ Full Assistance Special Instructions:	❑ Independent ❑ Partial Assistance ❑ Full Assistance Special Instructions:
WALKING	BLADDER FUNCTION
❑ Independent ❑ Partial Assistance ❑ Full Assistance Special Instructions:	❑ Continent (Full control) ❑ Partial Continence (Occasional mishaps) ❑ Incontinent (No control) Special Instructions:

MOVING AND POSITIONING	BOWEL FUNCTION
❏ Independent ❏ Partial Assistance ❏ Full Assistance Special Instructions:	❏ Continent (Full control) ❏ Partial Continence (Occasional mishaps) ❏ Incontinent (No control) Special Instructions:
VISION ❏ Full vision with or without correction ❏ Some to moderate difficulty ❏ Severe vision impairment Special Instructions: Describe any aides:	**COMMUNICATION** ❏ No impairment ❏ Partial impairment ❏ Full impairment/ Unable to convey needs Special Instructions:
HEARING ❏ Full hearing with or without aides ❏ Some to moderate difficulty ❏ Severe hearing impairment Special Instructions: Describe any aides:	**ENVIRONMENT/SAFETY MANAGEMENT** ❏ Independent ❏ Needs help to be safe ❏ Inability to manage environment for safety Special Instructions:

SLEEP PROBLEMS

❑ Never/rarely
❑ Sometimes (note triggers & solutions)
❑ Often (note triggers & solutions)

Special Bedtime Instructions:

BEHAVIOR

Pleasant/easy to get along with

Agitation/Aggressiveness

❑ Never
❑ Sometimes (note trigger & solution)
❑ Often (note trigger & solution)

Suspiciousness/Hostility

❑ Never
❑ Sometimes (note trigger & solution)
❑ Often (note trigger & solution)

Confusion/disorientation

❑ Never
❑ Sometimes (note trigger & solution)
❑ Often (note trigger & solution)

Wandering

❑ Never
❑ Sometimes (note trigger & solution)
❑ Often (note trigger & solution)

Repetitious questions

❑ Never
❑ Sometimes (note topics)
❑ Often (note usual response)

Special Instructions:

MEDICATION MANAGEMENT

❑ Independent
❑ Partial Assistance
❑ Full Assistance

Special Instructions:

Other considerations or special instructions (Stressors, Signs of Trouble and what to do about it):

_____

_____

_____

_____

_____

_____

_____

_____

_____

_____

_____

_____

_____

_____

_____

_____

_____

Instrumental Daily Living Skills
(Abilities and Assistance required)

USES TELEPHONE ❏ Independent ❏ Partial Assistance ❏ Full Assistance Special Instructions:	**LAUNDRY** ❏ Independent ❏ Partial Assistance ❏ Full Assistance Special Instruction
COOKING ❏ Independent ❏ Partial Assistance ❏ Full Assistance Special Instructions:	**SHOPPING** ❏ Independent ❏ Partial Assistance ❏ Full Assistance Special Instructions
HOUSEKEEPING ❏ Independent ❏ Partial Assistance or Needs supervision ❏ Full Assistance Special Instructions:	**USE OF STOVE** ❏ Uses safely ❏ Uses unsafely ❏ Does not use Special Instructions
TRANSPORTATION ❏ Independent/Drives self ❏ Uses public transportation ❏ Depends on others Special Instructions:	**BANKING** ❏ Independent/Does own banking ❏ Partial Assistance by… (see note) ❏ Banking done my another (see note) Special Instructions:

Other considerations or special instructions (Stressors, Signs of Trouble and what to do about it):

_____

_____

_____

_____

_____

_____

_____

_____

_____

_____

_____

_____

_____

_____

_____

_____

_____

Social/Recreational/Spiritual Needs
(Abilities and Assistance required)

GENERAL SOCIAL ACTIVITIES	**VISITORS**
❑ Independent/Attends outside activities ❑ Partial Assistance to attend outside activities ❑ Unwilling/not able to attend outside activities Special Instructions:	❑ Capable/welcomes visitors ❑ Partial Assistance needed for visitors ❑ Unwilling/not able to have visitors Special Instructions:
REGULAR GROUP ACTIVITIES Attends_____ Frequency_____ Day(s) of week _____ ❑ Independent/Attends on own ❑ Partial Assistance to attend (see notes) Special Instructions:	**REGULAR GROUP ACTIVITIES** Attends_____ Frequency_____ Day(s) of week _____ ❑ Independent/Attends on own ❑ Partial Assistance to attend (see notes) Special Instructions:
REGULAR GROUP ACTIVITIES Attends_____ Frequency_____ Day(s) of week _____ ❑ Independent/Attends on own ❑ Partial Assistance to attend (see notes) Special Instructions:	**REGULAR GROUP ACTIVITIES** Attends_____ Frequency_____ Day(s) of week _____ ❑ Independent/Attends on own ❑ Partial Assistance to attend (see notes) Special Instructions:

Other considerations or special instructions:

_____

_____

_____

_____

_____

_____

_____

_____

_____

_____

_____

_____

_____

_____

_____

_____

_____

*This information was updated on_____.

Medication List

This is a list of all medications your friend or loved one is taking including prescriptions, over the counter medications, vitamins, and supplements.

* For Over the Counter (OTC) medication, note date started under date prescribed column

MEDICATION NAME	DATE PRESCRIBED *OTC	DOSE	FREQUENCY	REASON	DATE DISCONTINUED

Medication Tracker

To document prescription as well as over the counter medications, vitamins, and supplements

DATE	TIME	MEDICATION	DOSE	RESULT/COMMENTS
Mar 20/22	0900	Ibuprophen 400 mg	1 tab	Headache subsided

Treatments and Therapies

TREATMENT	WHO DOES IT?	HOW OFTEN?	SPECIAL INSTRUCTIONS

Semi-annual and Annual Reminders and Follow ups:

DATE	WHO/WHERE	REASON

Daily Routines and Special Instructions
(Add any additional categories)

Date:

PERSONAL CARE	MEALS
Personal Care Dressing Bathing	Breakfast
Hydration Toileting Activities	Lunch
Evening Undressing/Ready for bed	Supper
Other/Notes:	

It is helpful to have notes and records about care in one place. Tracking sheets for daily activities and medications can keep information close at hand for easy retrieval when communicating with health care professionals and other family members. Here are two templates that may be useful or adapted to suit your specific needs.

Daily Notes

To document concerns, activities, questions, unusual problems

DATE	TIME	NOTES

Contacts and people who assist with health and care needs

In this section you might have some or all of the following listed:

- Physician
- Case Manager
- Pharmacist
- Home Care
- Other Service Providers who can help at last minute
- Placement Assessors (for Assisted Living or Long Term care Options)
- Day Program
- Hospital
- Pharmacy
- Other: (Please list)

PEOPLE WHO ASSIST (e.g., direct providers such as your physician, pharmacist, case manager, home care, therapists):

Contacts reviewed and updated on_____.

Name	
Why you would contact them:	

Phone	Day
	Evening
	Cell

Best way to contact:	
Helps with	
Address if necessary	

Name	
Why you would contact them:	

Phone	Day
	Evening
	Cell

Best way to contact:	
Helps with	
Address if necessary	

Name	
Why you would contact them:	

Phone	Day
	Evening
	Cell

Best way to contact:	
Helps with	

Address if necessary	

Name	
Why you would contact them:	

Phone	Day
	Evening
	Cell

Best way to contact:	
Helps with	

Address if necessary	

Name	
Why you would contact them:	

Phone	Day
	Evening
	Cell

Best way to contact:	
Helps with	

Address if necessary	

Name	
Why you would contact them:	

Phone	Day
	Evening
	Cell

Best way to contact:	
Helps with	

Address if necessary	

Name	
Why you would contact them:	

Phone	Day
	Evening
	Cell

Best way to contact:	
Helps with	

Address if necessary	

Name	
Why you would contact them:	

Phone	Day
	Evening
	Cell

Best way to contact:	
Helps with	

Address if necessary	

Question Tracker for follow up Medical Appointments

Sometimes concerns arise that are important but not urgent. This is a place to track what concerns you or the questions you have for the next follow up appointment.

DATE	FOR WHOM?	QUESTION OR CONCERN	HISTORY OR REASON

Health Care Decision-making, Legal, and Financial Matters

Health care decisions need due consideration. First, others providing care need to understand what to do in an emergency as well as any special instructions. Have you and or your friend or loved one discussed their wishes? Do you know what they want done in case they are incapacitated and cannot provider direction?

Deciding what one wants done towards the end of life of in the case of emergency are sensitive and personal. This section of The Care Book is not intended to tell you *what* to do regarding health decision-making, personal directives, or living in making these important decisions. I urge you to take steps to ensure wishes are known, made explicit to others, and kept up to date in writing.

Often family members may be involved in decision-making but not always. Everyone involved with caring and supporting the individual needs to know where to find directions and directives.

Do Not Resuscitate Orders

There are a few big questions to answer, what is to be done in case of emergency? What are an individual's views on support if they are incapacitated? Is there a need for a Do Not Resuscitate (DNR) Order? Where is it kept? No legal or medical directive is needed to provide all life supporting assistance, but it is needed when there are exceptions. You can ask your case manager or physician what documents are necessary to complete to have a DNR order in place if that is something that is desired.

Personal Directives/Advance Directives

Personal directives (PD) or Advance Directives [AD] sometimes used interchangeably to refer to the same thing. They are directions that specify what life sustaining or prolonging interventions someone wants done if they are incapacitated and cannot make the decision themselves typically due to an incurable illness or injury. A directive ought to note what is right for your loved one according to their wishes, medical procedures they want or do not want under which conditions, their substitute decision-maker, and they can be as detailed as they need it to be. A first step is having conversations about directions at end of life and who are the people that need to be involved.

Power of Attorney

Power of attorney (POA) is the appointment of an individual or individuals who will make health care decisions, or other legal or financial decisions when a person is incapable of making their own decisions. It may be a legal or financial advisor, but is often a family member or may be a close friend.

There are legal processes for both PDs and POAs, so please check with your jurisdiction and/or your legal counsel. Your legal counsel will often provide forms for both and you can easily find generic templates on the internet.

End of Life Care

Thinking about care, interventions, and the place for end of life care and death are significant matters that make a difference for both the person dying and the friends and family that will be, or want to be, with them. It can mean the difference between a wonderful or not-so-good experience. As in other care decisions and choices, there are no wrong answers, but rather what is right and good for the individual their caregiver, and other close members of their family. A good death can happen in a variety of places including home, hospice, long-term care centre and even in hospital. Planning and making wishes known are what matters.

Death is as much a part of life as birth. There are people who can help with planning and conversations if you want that, such as your physician, case manager, nurses, funeral directors, clergy if they are involved, and others who specialize in matters related to death and dying. There are individuals who take on a greater role with families and may even be with families through the death and dying process such as a death therapist or death doula. They key point is that talking about end of life and dying arc necessary conversations. If you are needing support in this area, a good place to start is with one of the professionals involved in your loved ones care.

Medical Assistance in Dying (MAiD)

Medical Assistance in Dying (MAiD) is becoming more widely available in several countries. It means that a person who meets specific criteria may access assistance to die when those criteria are met. A person may access MAiD when they determine they have intolerable suffering and meet certain legal conditions, that is conditions and criteria that are set within the law of their jurisdiction.

Language matters in this discussion and the term medical assistance in dying is Canada's legal term for assisted death. Historical terminology and language used in other contexts like euthanasia and physician-assisted suicide are not exactly they same terms. Briefly, both terms can be triggering for various reasons. Euthanasia is laden with historical trauma related of the anti-choice movement in Canada and often refers to ending an animals life with chemical assistance. Because in many jurisdictions nurse practitioners can also provide MAiD the term physician-assisted is no longer an accurate term.

If this is a topic you and your loved one wants to learn more about, I recommend you seek out the excellent resources available through your local hospice or palliative care association and speak with your physician, case manager or nurse. You can also find excellent information from resources to providers who offer MAiD in your jurisdiction through on-line websites such as dyingwithdignity.ca in Canada or compassionate choices. com in the United States. From there, you can make inquiries to access professionals with whom you can discuss the specifics of your situation, learn more about medically assisted dying, and investigate further. It is a process, and taking the time to think about end of life choices and have the right professionals to talk to matters.

Legal and Financial Matters

You can have directives as well as POAs for health care, legal, and financial matters. POAs may be the same person or different representatives for different areas. It is up to the individual, but the important point is to ensure they are in place and able as well as willing to carry out the tasks.

You might want to save copies of personal directives, power of attorneys, or special orders in this book or note here where each can be found.

DOCUMENT NAME	WHERE KEPT (NOTE ORIGINAL AND ANY COPIES)
Do Not Resuscitate	
Personal Directive	
Power of Attorney	
Will	
Other Document Name:	
Other Document Name:	
Other Document Name:	

Samples, Guidelines, and Jurisdictional Regulations

Samples and Guidelines for forms and procedures discussed in this section vary to a degree from one jurisdiction to the next. Regardless of what country, province or state you are in, there will be legal guidelines, policies, and perhaps even legislation. Because forms vary from place to place and time to time, it is best to either search on-line or ask for assistance and samples from the professionals involved in these matters with you. If you are looking on-line use search terms as procedures, templates, or guidelines for [WHATEVER YOU ARE SPECIFICALLY LOOKING FOR SUCH AS ADVANCED DIRECTIVES].

Advisors/Authorizers

Some of the people you might list here might include insurance companies, banker, lawyer, accountant, trustee, or guardian. Of course, not all of these will apply to everyone.

CONTACT FOR	NAME AND ADDRESS	TELEPHONE/EMAIL		PURPOSE
Banker		Work Phone		
		Cell Phone		
		Email		
Lawyer		Work Phone		
		Cell Phone		
		Email		
Accountant		Work Phone		
		Cell Phone		
		Email		
Power of Attorney		Work Phone		
		Cell Phone		
		Email		
Trustee		Work Phone		
		Cell Phone		
		Email		
Guardian		Work Phone		
		Cell Phone		
		Email		
Insurance Agent		Work Phone		
		Cell Phone		
		Email		

Primary or Main Caregiver		Work Phone	
		Cell Phone	
		Email	
Other:		Work Phone	
		Cell Phone	
		Email	
Other:		Work Phone	
		Cell Phone	
		Email	

This information was updated on_____.

Organizations and Future Supports

In this section, you might note things like:

- Home Care Providers,
- Assisted Living Options,
- Long Term Care Facilities,
- Aides to Daily Living and Equipment Suppliers, or
- Caregiver Support Groups and Associations* this might be generic or disease specific like the MS Society, local Alzheimer's Society and so on as many disease specific associations offer caregiver supports.

Organization			Organization		
What they offer:			What they offer:		
Contact	Name:		Contact	Name:	
	Number:			Number:	
	Email:			Email:	
Best way to contact:			Best way to contact:		
Other contacts			Other contacts		
Address if necessary			Address if necessary		

Organization	
What they offer:	

Contact	Name:
	Number:
	Email:

Best way to contact:	

Other contacts	

Address if necessary	

Organization	
What they offer:	

Contact	Name:
	Number:
	Email:

Best way to contact:	

Other contacts	

Address if necessary	

Organization	
What they offer:	

Contact	Name:
	Number:
	Email:

Best way to contact:	

Other contacts	

Address if necessary	

Organization	
What they offer:	

Contact	Name:
	Number:
	Email:

Best way to contact:	

Other contacts	

Address if necessary	

Seeking Help, Support and Care for a friend or loved one

(adopted from The Accidental Caregiver)

Advocating for yourself or your loved one simply means asking for what you need. But you need to know how to ask for something and where to go. Be open and honest with what you need and have your reasons prepared. The following sections are suggestions of things to keep in mind when you're looking for information, care, and support.

Where to look?

- Caregiver associations have dedicated staff to provide support, information, advocacy, and linkages for caregivers.
- Disease and Disability Specific Organizations focus on the needs of clients with specific conditions like the MS Society, Parkinson's society, Health, Spinal Cord Injury associations, Cerebral palsy association. Sometimes these organizations have supports specifically for caregivers of people with various conditions.
- Seniors Organizations. With many older people becoming caregivers Seniors centers often have programs, referral and information services, or services for caregivers.
- Health Department Information line. This might be an 811 or 211 service in your area. Here is where to look for social workers, case managers or home care. You can call the information line to get numbers for home care or other programs in your area. Home care is the department than does assessments to determine your eligibility for care in your home.
- For crisis support call a distress for crisis line. They are often a source of support and know where to direct you depending on your need. Many have a directory for various community services and supports.
- Financial benefits supports are available to caregivers depending on eligibility and your area may have a benefit center through your local state or provincial government.
- When you need help with information or advocacy many of the places listed above have people designated as caregiver advisors or system navigators. If this service is not offered to you ask if they have such a person.

Remember, communication is key to getting the right help. Knowing what language to use can help you get prompt action.

Starting Points—Some questions to ask your health care provider or physician

- Where can I find equipment like wheelchairs or walkers?
- Where do I look help in the home, like home care?
- Is there any support for me, like an organization for family caregivers?
- Where would I look for funding programs that might be available to help pay for equipment or supplies?

Further, be as specific as you can. Here are some suggestions:

- I am finding that the allotted time is not working for us.
- I am not able to [LIFT or INSERT THE SPECIFIC TASKS HERE] him anymore.
- I am physically and mentally exhausted and need a break.
- I need more care for the [EVENING or THE SPECIFIC TIME].
- I would like to change the time of day the caregiver comes.

Keeping Track

- Regardless of how you ask for something keep a written record for yourself. Document the date, who your talked to or left a message with, what your request was, and the result.
- Do you need to follow up? If they say they will follow up with you, ask for a due date and let them know that you will follow up shortly after that date if you haven't received any feedback or action.
- You may feel like a nuisance, however, this can save you steps later if you don't get what you need right away. A paper trail can help you get action if your request goes unanswered for days or weeks on end. Having accurate information at your fingertips will let others know you are organized, competent, and determined to get your needs met. It is harder to defer someone who is ready with detailed information than someone who can't recall details such as who they last talked to, when, and the details of the conversation.

How to ask for what you need

Be direct, clear, and polite. Be open about what you need and why. Although it is not your problem, many of the people you will be seeking out are busy and possibly overworked. While they should be there for you, the client or the customer, in reality they likely have multiple people they are talking to and assisting so make things easy for them.

Most of us want to work with people who are kind, so don't underestimate politeness regardless of what you get back in return. If someone isn't helpful you can bring your request to their supervisor if needed, but first try your best to get what you need on your first call.

Regarding home care, your Case Manager is usually your main contact and they are in a position to help you get the care you need. If you do not feel heard despite repeated requests, or you don't feel understood, then it is time to take it further. Their supervisor, the supervisor's supervisor who might be a Team Leader or the Director of the Home Care Program is your next stop. If you don't feel comfortable doing that then organizations that support Caregivers can help. Places like Caregiver associations, eldercare, or even a Patient Advocate might exist within your area.

Finding support in your own community

Most families don't want a swinging door of service providers It can seem like an invasion of your space and your privacy. However, the right services at the right time can be a life saver. But you need accurate and current information to help you make the best choices. You can look for supports in person, by walking in to organizations or on the telephone or online. Here are some first steps:

In-person

Access a transition worker at your local health unit. **Case managers, social workers, or community resource specialists** can help you find the right resources in your own community. The individuals who can help you are called different things so ask who is available to help you find resources to help you care for your loved one.

Then ask questions like:

Do you have any print information on various programs I can take with me? What does each program offer? How do I access it? What is the phone number? Who is the best person to talk to?

If you or your loved one are an older person, ask about local organizations that provide programs and services for older people. Ask friends who work in health care where you can find information. Don't be shy. Ask your physician or a nurse in the doctor's office and hospital. If they don't know, then push them to look into it for you while you wait. Look up "Home Care" or "Community Care."

Once you connect with a good resource, you will likely find it easier to get referred to others for information and support.

Home Care Programs

Formal organizations that may either be private home care companies or Government home programs provide care workers. Sometimes government programs both authorize and provide the care directly with their own employees and other times they assess needs and authorize another organization on the type and amount of care to provide. Private home care companies offer care either through government programs or insurance, or directly to clients on a fee for service basis.

Typically care is provided by an unlicensed person who is educated to provide personal care or by licensed nurses who may either be a licensed practical nurse (LPN) or registered Nurse (RN). Rehabilitation specialists such as physical therapists or occupational therapists may also be providing support. **Personal care assistants or health care aides**–they are called by different titles in different jurisdictions—have a short education (usually 306 months) and are unregulated. **Nurse**s are regulated professionals. Different home care programs provide different levels of service. Who provides your care depends on what you need, based on a thorough assessment that usually takes 60-90 minutes.

The **assessment** may be carried out by a regulated health care professional, usually a nurse but could be a social worker or a rehabilitation professional. They may be called a **Case Manager**. Think about where you need help to care for your loved one and ask for the support you need.

Some questions to ask are:

What kinds of care providers are available? Is there a cost? What kinds of things can I get help with?

Ask about things like personal care such as bathing, dressing, toileting. What about meal preparation or feeding? What about laundry?

Can I break up the amount of time I am eligible for? What makes us eligible for home care? Can I get care at night-time? What about respite so I can leave the home without worrying? How many times a week can I get that?

Are Private services available? If I want more than is provided by the government home care program can I "top up" by purchasing private care? What private home care companies are in the area? Do you have any information on them? Do they also work with home care?

In many jurisdictions, home care is contracted by the public (government) home care program to private service provider agencies who employ health care aides and personal care attendants and in some cases the nurses. What the public program contracts out varies by jurisdiction. The private service providers under government contract, have to prove they meet specific standards. This is usually done by various reporting and auditing regulations by the contracting government agency.

Online Information

The accessibility of information caregivers can access has improved with the internet, but the quality of the material you unearth will depend on your ability to search well, so being somewhat internet savvy and having a little bit of knowledge about what to look for can help. Some of the information in this book is a good start.

A single comprehensive website targeted to family caregivers and regularly updated would be a fantastic resource, but information is often found in different places. However, there are organizations that exist solely to support caregivers, and they usually have good websites. As well, most programs and services will have a websites, and many link to other community supports and on-line resources.

Search terms you might try:

- Family caregiving in [my neighbourhood or city]
- Supports for
- Resources for
- Home care program
- Supports for seniors

- Home care
- Meal program
- Meal delivery
- Services for care at home
- Private home care
- Home support services
- Home health care equipment
- Home care supplies

The terms home health, home care, home support might all yield different results but are terms that are sometimes used interchangeably.

Be aware of the publisher of the site you are looking at. Is it the organizations own site or a third party site promoting something? Is it a government site? A good tip is that the organizations name or the government will actually appear in their web name.

Regardless of where you are on your caregiving journey, do your best to be organized, create a system that works as you may hear about supports that you don't need now but that may be helpful down the road.

Templates/Forms

Please make additional copies these forms as you need them. Some caregivers start a binder and three hole punch the pages and keep them in order by section. You can find dividers at your local office supply store. Other people find it helpful keep them in a file folder. An important consideration is to date each page so you can keep them in order, noting dates when information is updated. This is especially helpful when you want to recall aspects of care and activities.

If you would like digital copies of the Templates used in The Care Book, please visit www.kimberlyfraserauthor.com and request a downloadable version of The Templates used in The Care Book.

Daily Schedule At-a-Glance

AM _____

_____

_____

NOON _____

_____

_____

PM _____

_____

_____

EVENING _____

_____

_____

Notes: _____

_____

_____

_____

_____

_____

_____

Weekly Schedule At-a-Glance

TIME (AM/PM)	MON	TUES	WED	THURS	FRI	SAT	SUN

Notes: _____

_____

_____

_____

_____

_____

*This information was updated on_____.

Daily Routines and Special Instructions
(Add any additional categories)

Date:

PERSONAL CARE	MEALS
Personal Care Dressing Bathing	Breakfast
Hydration Toileting Activities	Lunch
Evening Undressing/Ready for bed	Supper
Other/Notes:	

Daily Notes

To document concerns, activities, questions, unusual problems

DATE	TIME	NOTES

Medication List

MEDICATION NAME	DOSE	FREQUENCY	REASON	DATE DISCONTINUED

Medication Tracker

To document prescription as well as over the counter medications, vitamins, and supplements

DATE	TIME	MEDICATION	DOSE	RESULT/COMMENTS

Treatments and Therapies

TREATMENT	DATE STARTED	WHO DOES IT?	HOW OFTEN?	SPECIAL INSTRUCTIONS/ DATE DISCONTINUED

Question Tracker
(for follow ups at medical appointments)

Sometimes concerns arise that are important but not urgent. This is a place to track what concerns you or the questions you have for the next follow up appointment.

DATE	WHO FOR?	QUESTION OR CONCERN	HISTORY OR REASON

People who Assist

Last updated _____.

Name		Name	
Why you would contact them:		Why you would contact them:	
Phone	Day	Phone	Day
	Evening		Evening
	Cell		Cell
Best way to contact:		Best way to contact:	
Helps with		Helps with	
Address if necessary		Address if necessary	
Name		Name	
Why you would contact them:		Why you would contact them:	
Phone	Day	Phone	Day
	Evening		Evening
	Cell		Cell
Best way to contact:		Best way to contact:	
Helps with		Helps with	
Address if necessary		Address if necessary	

Name	
Why you would contact them:	

Phone	Day
	Evening
	Cell

Best way to contact:	
Helps with	
Address if necessary	

Name	
Why you would contact them:	

Phone	Day
	Evening
	Cell

Best way to contact:	
Helps with	
Address if necessary	

Name	
Why you would contact them:	

Phone	Day
	Evening
	Cell

Best way to contact:	
Helps with	
Address if necessary	

Name	
Why you would contact them:	

Phone	Day
	Evening
	Cell

Best way to contact:	
Helps with	
Address if necessary	

Name	
Why you would contact them:	

Phone	Day
	Evening
	Cell

Best way to contact:	
Helps with	
Address if necessary	

Name	
Why you would contact them:	

Phone	Day
	Evening
	Cell

Best way to contact:	
Helps with	
Address if necessary	

Glossary and Meaning of Terms you hear when you are a caregiver

Activities of Daily Living (ADLs): daily personal care tasks that people do to manage their physical needs. They either do these activities for themselves or have others partially or fully assist them such as toileting, bathing, dressing, eating, and (ambulating) moving about.

Aids to Daily Living programs: a community resource that offered supplies and equipment for care in the home. The supplies and equipment may be offered for free, on loan, or for a fee. The Alberta Aids to Daily Living Program is one example and is commonly referred to in Alberta as the **AADL program** (Alberta Aids to Daily Living).

Assisted Living/Supportive Living: A building or group of buildings in a space where varying levels of care are available. People may choose to live in one of these settings before they are ill or infirm with the intent of staying there until death. There are varying levels and varying costs. Services may include meal programs, in-home care or assistance, cleaning, hair stylists, exercise and activity programs and some even offer long-term care in designated sections.

Care Coordinator: May be similar to the case manager but this person may also be the scheduling person in a home care provider agency.

Care Provider: Someone who is paid for caregiving. They may work for an organization or be paid directly by the family. They are either in a regulated position such as a nurse or rehabilitation professional or a non-regulated position such as a health care aide.

Case Manager: assesses and plans care the client will receive in home care. They are often the first point of contact and the family caregivers main contact for the home care program. In some areas they may be called a care manager, care coordinator, or case coordinator. They may act as the main coordinator for communication with the client, family, care provider agency, physicians, or other community providers.

Client: a person who receives care, therapies, or treatments. Often called a client in home and community care.

Family Caregiver: Family caregivers provide care and support to a loved one who may or may not be receiving care from home care or live in a care facility such as a long term care home or an assisted living facility. There may be several family caregivers or friends who support an individual but often there is one primary family caregiver

Fragmented (system): lack of collaboration or any relationship between departments and agencies.

Health Care Aide/Personal Care Aide/Home Health Aide: are a non-regulated care provider that may work directly for the Home Care Program or through a service provider agency that a family hires. Sometimes they work independently rather than through an organization and are hired directly by families. They typically receive eight to 16 weeks of training in personal care, either through an educational institution or through an employer. There are several terms used for this level of care provider. In this book I use care provider when referring to any paid personnel.

Home Care/Home Health Care: Home care programs may be private, not-for-profit or government run organizations. In this book Home Care is usually referencing a government home care program that is available in all provinces and territories in Canada. The actual services may be provided directly by the government program or through a private or not for profit agency under contract. Clients and families may also purchase services privately or costs may be covered by a third party such as an insurance provider. In the US, Home care may be covered by Medicare or Medicaid but is most often through a private or not for profit organization.

Instrumental Activities of Daily Living (IADLs): necessary activities that require more complex thinking and organizational skills but that do not involve personal care. These include things such as transportation, cooking, shopping, banking and buying groceries.

Long Distance Caregiver: Family caregiver(s) who do not live in the same geographic region as the client who needs care. They may be the designated contact or caregiver when care is provided by a home care program or in a long term care home. The **California Daughter Syndrome** is a colloquial term that refers to a family caregiver who is often not directly involved in day to day caregiving or care decisions, yet when they come to town the often enter the caregiving scene with a flurry of activity and opinion about the caregiving and needs of their loved one whether or not there is a family caregiver engaged as the primary contact and caregiver.

Long-term care home: A residential facility where care is provided to clients. They may be called care home, nursing home, continuing care home, or extended care home.

Patient: a person who receives care, therapies, or treatments. Often called a patient in hospital based care and physician clinics.

Registered Nurse/Licensed Practical Nurse/Registered Psychiatric Nurse: A **nurse** is a regulated professional with two to five years of basic nursing education depending on their title and education program. They are regulated by a licensing body through which the nurse has annual registration and competency requirements in order to receive provincial or state licensure to work in many health care settings.

Respite Care: Care provided to the client but for the benefit of the family caregiver. **In-home respite** is provided by a paid care provider to a client in the home and the family may or may not receive other kinds of home care services. **Out-of-home respite** is provided in a setting other than the home and is designed to give the family caregiver a longer break from caregiving such as a weekend, a few weeks, or perhaps as long as a month. Settings for out of home respite may be designated beds in a long term care home, an assisted living environment, or even in a hospital in some instances.

Siloed (system): a system where people work within closed environments–often completely unaware or ignorant to other parts that are equally closed off, making communication and coordination virtually impossible. Fragmented and siloed systems affect comprehensive service delivery and often lead to inconsistencies or redundancies, both can have negative impacts on both quality and safety of care for clients and families.

Support Worker, Respite Worker, or Companion Sitter: typically would not provide any hands-on care but may do light housekeeping, meal prep, but not feeding, and companionship and leisure.

About the Author

DR. KIMBERLY FRASER is an author, speaker, and former Associate Professor at the Faculty of Nursing with the University of Alberta, and Clinician Scientist-Home Care with Alberta Health Services. She now does part-time contract teaching at Athabasca University and devotes most of her time to writing and community board work.

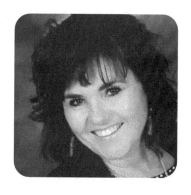

Kim writes about family caregiving, home care, and related health policy. Her book, *The Accidental Caregiver: Wisdom and guidance for the unexpected challenges of family caregiving* is available through Sutherland House Books or your local bookstore.

Kim provides talks and workshops on family caregiving and healthy aging. You can find out more or contact Kim at www.kimberlyfraserauthor.com.